How to De-Stress in Five Minutes a Day

Inspiring Ideas to Help You Unwind Every Day

JOANNE MALLON

vie

HOW TO DE-STRESS IN FIVE MINUTES A DAY

An Hachette UK Company
www.hachette.co.uk

Vie Books, an imprint of Summersdale Publishers
Part of Octopus Publishing Group Limited
Carmelite House
50 Victoria Embankment
LONDON
EC4Y 0DZ
UK

This FSC® label means that materials and other controlled sources used for the product have been responsibly sourced

MIX
Paper | Supporting responsible forestry
FSC® C016973
www.fsc.org

www.summersdale.com

The authorized representative in the EEA is Hachette Ireland, 8 Castlecourt Centre, Dublin 15, D15 XTP3, Ireland (email: info@hbgi.ie)

Printed and bound in China

ISBN: 978-1-83799-743-5
eISBN: 978-1-83799-744-2

Disclaimer
Neither the author nor the publisher can be held responsible for any injury, loss or claim – be it health, financial or otherwise – arising out of the use, or misuse, of the suggestions made herein. This book is not intended as a substitute for the medical advice of a doctor or physician. If you are experiencing problems with your physical or mental health, it is always best to follow the advice of a medical professional.

Contents

Introduction

Let's face it, life is stressful. But we are strong and can handle it. Small amounts of stress can even be a good thing - the deadline that helps you get work done; the excitement of starting a new job or project; the fun of visiting somewhere new. But too much stress can be overwhelming, and if left unchecked, can lead to physical and mental illness. Learning to deal with stress will reduce this negative impact and boost your everyday well-being.

This book will help you rise above everyday stresses, becoming more resilient and able to cope when the big stuff hits. It takes you through a day in your life, with suggestions for antidotes to stress that will work in the morning, daytime and evening, as well as longer lasting solutions to support you in the future. Everything is designed to be achievable in 5 minutes or less, and slot easily into your life. Feel free to adapt any of these tips, or use them as inspiration for an idea of your own.

You may not be able to completely eliminate the stress in your life, but with these tips you'll learn to rise above it and stop stress dragging you down.

You have power over your mind – not outside events. Realize this, and you will find strength.

MARCUS AURELIUS

CHAPTER ONE:

Stress-Free Mornings

How you spend your morning sets the tone for the day ahead. The tips in this chapter will help you create a morning that's smoother, calmer and a great place from which to ease into your day. Taking the stress out of your mornings will benefit you long into the afternoon and evening.

Read through this section and commit to following at least one tip for the next week. Pick the one that resonates most or seems to fit the most easily into your day. Add it to your routine alongside something you already do out of habit, such as taking a shower or having breakfast.

Get ahead of the stress

Stress is one way our body reacts to the challenges life places on it. Before your day gets going, ask yourself: What do I expect to be the most challenging part of today?

Is there a project that needs to be completed, a difficult conversation that needs to be had or a task you'd rather avoid? Making a plan and breaking down these challenges into manageable chunks will help you feel more in control. Deciding what to do in advance (either through journalling, rehearsing a conversation or simply thinking through your day) will help you deal with your daily stressors more easily.

What you do every day matters more than what you do once in a while.

GRETCHEN RUBIN

First rise

A morning routine that rushes from one thing to another is a stressful way to start the day, so give yourself the gift of a few extra minutes for self-care. Aim to be the first person awake in your home and you'll get to enjoy a calming break before the day gets going. You may even want to get up early enough to enjoy the quiet awe of a sunrise. Move with intention before life gets a chance to become overwhelming. Step outside to get a little morning sunlight on your face. Clear your mind before it gets bogged down.

Look for the little joys

Spend a few moments thinking about the bright sparks that will illuminate your path today. What are you most looking forward to? What's good about today? Capture the joy by writing down whatever comes to mind. It could be something small like a delicious lunch or something bigger such as fun with friends. These tiny sparks of joy are what make tougher, messier times easier to deal with. Psychologists have found that anticipation can actually be more enjoyable than doing the thing itself, so by anticipating the joys of the day, you'll get double the benefit.

Morning meditation

Many scientific studies have found that meditation is one of the most effective ways to reduce stress. Even 1 or 2 minutes of meditation a day can help reset a busy mind, so start small and you'll immediately feel the benefits. Simply sit in a quiet spot, close your eyes and focus on your breath as it moves in and out. It's fine if your mind wanders – it probably will. Just keep coming back to the breath until it feels natural to open your eyes again. A little morning meditation will help you start your day with a clear, calm and focused mind.

Try morning pages

A morning brain dump into your journal can be a really effective way to get a handle on all the stress in your life. A few minutes of scribbling down your thoughts will help you process any stress that's currently whirring around your mind. Take those worries out of your head and put them on the page where they won't feel quite so overwhelming. Don't stop to think as you write – just put your pen to paper and get it all out. Your troubles will become more manageable once they're out of your head and down on paper.

ACT FOR TODAY,
AS IF LIFE HAS YOUR
BACK COMPLETELY.

DONNA LANCASTER

Pay attention to your first hour

To feel calmer and less stressed every day, focus on the first hour you're awake in the morning. Our levels of cortisol – the stress hormone – are at their highest when we first wake up. Scientists call this the cortisol awakening response (CAR). It's experienced by around 77 per cent of adults and is regarded as part of our body's natural daily rhythm. CAR helps us wake up and have energy to face the day. But if you're already stressed, this can worsen the effects of CAR.

How do you spend the first hour of your day right now? What's the first thing you look at when you open your eyes? Is it a loved one, a calm environment – or is it your phone? This is the time when calming activities will bring significant benefit, so use them wisely. Stretch; breathe; move with purpose. Drink a glass of water slowly; step outside and gaze at the sky.

If you often feel stressed and anxious first thing in the morning, CAR could be a factor. Set an intention to stay away from your phone for the first hour you're awake. This will probably mean charging it outside your bedroom and using something else as an alarm clock.

Make your morning drink a ritual

Take time to savour your first drink of the day, whether it's a matcha latte or a simple glass of water. Use your favourite mug or glass that fits well in your hand. Make your drink exactly how you like it. Sit somewhere comfortable and quiet to relax. Take a brief pause in order to energize before the stressors of the day have a chance to bite. Find calm in this small moment.

Shake it off

Studies show that upbeat music, accompanied by movement, can reduce activity in the amygdala (a part of the brain linked to anxiety) and increase the release of the "reward hormone" dopamine. It can also help lower cortisol levels, leading to a reduction in feelings of anxiety. In a nutshell, dancing makes us feel good. Soundtrack the start of your day with your favourite upbeat banger and give it your best moves. You could put on a joyful playlist to pump up your morning, or take 3 minutes to dance to your favourite pop song before you sit down to work.

Design a de-stress breakfast

Your first meal of the day has the power to fuel you calmly if you get smart about what it contains. Aim to include nutrients that will help regulate your mood and stabilize blood sugar and you'll feel the benefits for the rest of the day. Prioritize protein, as it contains amino acids, which help the brain produce neurotransmitters that manage our mood. You could try:

- Bananas – contain potassium and B6 vitamins to boost serotonin.
- Nuts (particularly almonds and walnuts) – good source of protein and fibre.

- Oats (in the form of muesli, porridge or overnight oats) – high in fibre, which will stabilize your blood sugar and prevent energy crashes later in the day. They're a good source of protein, higher than most other grains.
- Spinach – contains magnesium, which helps reduce stress. Add it to an omelette or smoothie.

Other breakfast foods with great stress-busting properties include avocados, chia seeds, eggs and Greek yoghurt. You could combine some of these ingredients in a smoothie for a maximum morning-vitamin blast.

Anxiety happens when you think you have to figure out everything all at once. Breathe. You're strong. You got this.

KAREN SALMANSOHN

Be caffeine-wise

Scientists say that the best time to have coffee is between 9.30 a.m. and 11.30 a.m., as this is when it will help boost energy without interfering with the body's natural circadian rhythm. However, too much caffeine can contribute to stress by overstimulating us, raising cortisol levels and interfering with sleep. Remember that "decaf" doesn't always mean "no caf", so go easy on decaffeinated drinks. Be mindful and intentional with your morning coffee. Use it to lift you, not stress you. Listen to your body to find that sweet spot, where caffeine is supporting you rather than draining you.

Stress is caused
by being “here” but
wanting to be “there”.

ECKHART TOLLE

Dress to de-stress

Clothes have a big impact on how we feel. Hence the term "dopamine dressing" – dressing in a way that gives you a feel-good hit.

Psychologists have found that yellow and orange are particularly positive colours, green and blue can make us feel calmer and more serene, while red is stimulating. As you choose your clothes this morning, dress mindfully by thinking about how you want to feel today. If wearing bright colours isn't your thing, that's fine. Wear what you love and what makes you feel good. Let your clothing lift you up and bring you joy.

Inhale calm

Certain scents have been shown to help reduce stress, promote relaxation and improve mood. In the morning, there are many easy ways to surround yourself with stress-relieving aromas, such as using perfume, moisturizer, body oil, shower gel, a diffuser, a scented candle, herbal tea or even in your choice of washing powder.

The most effective scents for stress relief are:

- Bergamot – often used in aromatherapy to improve emotional well-being.
- Camomile – can reduce anxiety and soothe the mind.
- Citrus – scents such as orange and lemon can be great energizing mood boosters. Look for them in household products.
- Jasmine – often used in aromatherapy to calm nerves, reduce anxiety and promote a sense of peace.
- Lavender – calming and soothing, can be used day or night.
- Peppermint – refreshing and great for digestion. Apply a few drops of peppermint oil to your temples to clear your mind.
- Rose – this sweet, floral scent is known to reduce anxiety and promote emotional healing.

It's okay to pace yourself, get a little rest, and speak of your struggles out loud. It's okay to prioritize your wellness.

MICHELLE OBAMA

Ground yourself with a mantra

If you could sum up your expectations for today in a word or a phrase, what would it be? What do you want today to stand for?

A mantra is a short, positive word or phrase, like "om", repeated either silently or aloud. It can ground you, relax you and give you something positive to focus on – similar to a breathing exercise but with added sound. You can create your own mantra by thinking about how you want to feel today.

Here are some words to inspire you:

- Breathe
- Calm
- Happy
- Safe
- Peace

Just breathe

Breathing exercises work by switching on the parasympathetic nervous system (the one that tells your brain there's no threat, also known as "rest and digest"). There are lots of different breathing exercises to try, but the main thing to remember is to breathe in slowly through the nose, pause for a moment or two, then breathe out through the mouth. The great thing about using the breath to feel calmer is that it's easy, and you always have your breath with you. If you start to feel stressed this morning, deep, slow breaths will calm you down within seconds.

BREATHE OUT NEGATIVITY. BREATHE IN RELAXATION. BREATHE OUT STRESS.

GARY MACK

Pause for a pet

Pets are great for de-stressing and emotional support. Petting an animal releases oxytocin (the "love hormone"), making us feel more relaxed and less stressed. You can benefit from this feeling even if you don't have a pet, by spending time around animals whenever you get the chance. If you do have a pet, you'll know they love us unconditionally for who we are (though they might not show it if they're a cat). If you have a little furry friend, they're probably already looking for your attention in the morning – we don't have a choice in that matter! So, take your time. Enjoy the moment of connection and unconditional love.

Caring for your pet provides structure to your day. If you have a dog, there's a need to go outside for a walk even on days when you might not feel like it. Like anything that we do every day, we might not appreciate the support and love we get from our pets. Make a point of pausing for a moment to say good morning to your best animal friend. Give them a stroke, ask them how they are, and tell them how you're doing today.

You don’t have to see
the whole staircase,
just take the first step.

MARTIN LUTHER KING JR

Try yoga

Yoga has been helping people de-stress for thousands of years. Its combination of movement, breathwork and mindfulness will make you feel calmer very quickly. Morning yoga is particularly good for gently stretching and waking up the body, relieving any stiffness you might have accumulated while you were asleep. If you're new to yoga, check out the many free YouTube channels dedicated to the practice. Try a "cat-cow" exercise to stretch the spine or a "downward dog pose" to wake up the muscles. Take 5 minutes to stretch and simply be aware of your body.

Cold exposure

Cold water is a shock to the system, but a positive one! Splashing cold water on your face or wrists, or taking a cold shower, can activate the parasympathetic response, particularly through the vagus nerve. The vagus nerve carries signals from the brain to the body and helps us feel calmer after a stressful episode. It particularly helps the body get out of "fight or flight" mode. Consider beginning your day by either jumping straight into cold water, or easing yourself into it by standing under the shower as the water warms up.

Optimistic fuel

Start your day by learning something new and positive. This will help you see the possibilities in your future as you open your mind. Choose to read a few pages of a book, listen to an audiobook or tune in to a positive podcast. Look beyond the traditional news sources, which can sometimes feel a little doom and gloom. Instead, take in optimistic fuel to help expand your mind and ensure that you face today on an upwards course. Give 5 minutes to positivity and take yourself somewhere new.

CHAPTER TWO:

Stress-Free Days

No day is ever 100 per cent predictable. Life is full of curveballs, plot twists and surprises. And it is this uncertainty that can lead to stress, as our brains crave predictability to feel safe. The tips in this chapter are designed to help you deal with this, however, and wherever, you spend your day.

Is there a particular part of your day that tends to add the most stress? Commit to trying a couple of these ideas over the coming week and let them take you to a more peaceful place.

Embrace uncertainty today

It's the uncertainty in life that can lead to stress, and the solution lies in relying on yourself to handle whatever today brings. Pause a moment to remind yourself – you've got this. Be at peace with the unexpected. Know that you can handle whatever today has in store.

The world is not going to stop being uncertain, therefore the only thing we can change is the attitude we bring to it. Try to ride the waves rather than letting them pull you under. Stop looking to be in control because that is, after all, impossible. Practise acceptance and embrace uncertainty today.

Make a choice, right now, to be guided by challenges that you may face instead of being put off by them.

ROXIE NAFOUSI

The 20/20/20 technique

If your day involves a lot of screen time, the 20/20/20 technique is a great, quick way to give your mind and body regular breaks and insert some balance into your life.

It's a simple method that was invented by an optometrist to help reduce eye strain and stop screen users from getting too stressed. Here's how it works:

- Every 20 minutes, take a break from looking at your screen. Use an alarm on your phone to remind you, or keep a sand timer on your desk.

- As you break from looking at the screen, look at something 20 feet away (around 6 metres – the length of one and a half cars) for at least 20 seconds.
- Use the break to take a drink of water, stretch, close your eyes or do anything else that will give your eyes and mind a rest. This isn't the time to start checking your phone.

Using this technique of short, regular breaks will stop stress from building and taking hold, and help you focus more effectively when you get back to work.

You see only the beautiful things when you stand still.

HEATHER O'NEILL

Listen to the birds

In prehistoric times, hearing birdsong meant that everything was safe and there were no predators around. This association persists in the primitive part of our brain. That's why we feel safer, calmer and less stressed when we hear birds – it's a sign that all is well. Step outside for a moment today and tune your ears in to the calming songs of nature.

Play with stress-relief toys

Stress-relief toys such as squishy balls, fidget spinners or soft toys can be useful to keep on your desk or in your pocket/bag to help you cope with stress in the moment and prevent overwhelm. They provide a way to release physical tension and can also aid in concentration and focus. They're especially useful when you're in an online meeting as you can hold them in your hand discreetly. Plus they can be cute, fun and make you smile. Stress-relief toys are for all ages, so pick one to play with today.

Looking towards joy is the most important part of rewiring the stress response.

MIRANDA HART

Try a tech-free lunch

Make your midday break an actual break by switching off from technology while you have your meal. Put your phone in a drawer. Focus on your food and enjoy it. Savour the flavours mindfully. Chat to others if they're around. Be fully present and focused, without your phone calling for your attention. You might even be inspired to expand this for a longer digital retreat, by going out for a walk and leaving your devices behind.

Adopt a tree

Studies have found that spending time in nature lowers cortisol levels, making it a great way to de-stress. Why not choose a tree in your local environment and pay special attention to how it changes each time you see it. Think of it as your pet tree. Adopting it will help maintain perspective, as it encourages your mind to focus on the bigger picture. Notice how it might blossom in spring, bloom in summer, change colour in autumn, stand bare in winter and then repeat the cycle again. Your adopted tree will help you appreciate the broader story of life and feel grounded.

Complete a snack workout

Physical movement will trigger the release of endorphins ("feel-good" hormones) and keep you lifted long after you've finished exercising. However, it can be a challenge to fit a full workout into a busy day. So how about a little "snack" workout instead?

Five-minute "movement snacks" are brief, targeted bursts of activity. You could walk outside after lunch, do some squats while the kettle's boiling, or fit in a few lunges, gentle backbends, stretches, push-ups or planks. All these exercises can be effective, even if you only do them for a few minutes. Alternatively, you could aim to walk faster or jog every time you have to go up or down the stairs. Try elevated push-ups, with your hands on the edge of your desk or sofa, or up the intensity with a high-intensity interval training (HIIT) workout. Check YouTube for lots of ideas around quick-exercise snack workouts and aim to do one every day this week.

Realize that stress doesn't happen because the world has made some pact against you personally.

JIM BRICKMAN

Give yourself a hand massage

Our hands work hard *for* us and can pick up a lot of tension throughout the day. Massaging them will stimulate pressure points, reducing physical tension and encouraging the release of endorphins. Warm your hands by rubbing them together to help the blood flow and reduce muscle tension. You can double up on the relaxing effect of massage by using an oil or lotion with a calming scent. Spend a few moments now giving love and attention to your precious hands.

Daily creativity

Being creative involves concentrating on what you're doing and nothing else in that moment, making creativity a fantastic mindfulness de-stressor.

Your daily creative practice could be writing, drawing or painting, or it could be cooking, gardening or simply dressing in a certain way. It could be something tiny – a line of lipstick, a random doodle, a quick poem. It doesn't matter what you create. This exercise is all about the journey and allowing yourself to make space for creativity. It's the process of reconnecting with yourself by giving yourself freedom – freedom to play, to express yourself, to relax.

If you can make it easier, make it easier, and don't feel guilty about it.

ALI WONG

The power of affirmations

While affirmations have existed for centuries, in the 1980s, social psychologists began researching how positive affirmations could rewire our subconscious thought patterns. Although they are similar in some ways to one-word mantras, an affirmation tends to be a complete sentence that references a goal as if we already achieved it.

So, you could say:

- **I am calm and at peace. I am enough.**
- **I am full of love and compassion today.**
- **I am safe and well and everything is okay.**
- **I am letting go of my worries and breathing in calm.**
- **I trust myself to handle whatever today brings.**

Choose an affirmation that resonates with you and repeat it every day. The more you say it, the more you will believe it. You could also write it down in your journal or combine your affirmation with deep breathing or a meditation practice.

DON'T EVER DOUBT YOURSELVES OR WASTE A SECOND OF YOUR LIFE. IT'S TOO SHORT, AND YOU'RE TOO SPECIAL.

ARIANA GRANDE

Observe your stress to make it less

As you go through today, notice where the major moments of stress are coming from. Aim to be slightly detached, observing those moments like a scientist in a laboratory. Doing this creates emotional distance, as if you are mentally standing back from the stress, which will help you manage it more effectively. Is today's stress what you thought it might be? How many of these stressors happening today can you do something about? If you can change them, do. If you can't, let them go. Ask yourself – what needs to be different here?

Move with *qigong*

Qigong (pronounced "chee-gong") is a gentle type of movement, like a more dynamic form of tai chi. Any kind of movement is great for dealing with stress, but *qigong* is particularly effective because of its combination of gentle moves, focused breathing and mental relaxation.

The name refers to *qi* (energy) and *gong* (work). It involves working with the body's natural energy to improve health and well-being. The slow, deliberate movements help the body relax and activate the parasympathetic nervous system. You'll find many 5-minute *qigong* routines on YouTube, so, why not give it a try?

Take a mindful pause

Stop what you're doing right now. Close your eyes and pause to check in with your body. How are you feeling, both emotionally and physically? Are you aware of any tension in your body? Out of ten, how calm do you feel? If it's not a ten, what (if anything) would have to change to make it so?

Pausing to check in with yourself will catch any stress that's rising, and remind you when life is good.

Stay hydrated

Drinking a glass of water is one of the quickest and easiest things we can do to reduce stress. Staying hydrated is an important part of stress management, as the body produces more cortisol when it's dehydrated, and this can lead to feelings of stress and anxiety. As well as helping you stay hydrated, water is good for mental clarity, balancing blood pressure and improving sleep quality. Keep water bottles wherever you spend most time – on your work desk, in your gym bag, in the kitchen. In addition, aim to include hydrating foods in your diet, such as watermelon and cucumber.

What mental health needs is more sunlight, more candor, and more unashamed conversation.

GLENN CLOSE

Be kind to others

Scientific research has proven that doing kind acts for others can help reduce stress and make us feel more positive. This is known as the "helper's high" – a boost we get when we do something good for somebody else, whether that's a favour for a friend, holding a door open for a stranger or volunteering. All these things will reduce cortisol and boost the release of feel-good hormones such as oxytocin and serotonin.

Helping others shifts our focus away from our own situation, however stressful that may be, and out into the wider world. It's good to feel needed, and part of a community. Social connections are strengthened as a result. We feel better about ourselves as we see that we have something good to give to the world. So, look for a way, however small, to be kind to someone else today. Smile and say thank you. Be generous with your time and attention. Help others and you'll help yourself too.

A daily square of dark chocolate

Dark chocolate (70 per cent cocoa or higher) has been found to have stress-relieving benefits. It's rich in magnesium, which helps regulate the nervous system, and contains compounds that will boost serotonin and release endorphins. Dark chocolate also includes antioxidants, which help reduce inflammation and protect the body from stress. In moderation, it's practically a health food, so enjoy!

Draw a line under the work of today

At the end of your working day, clear your desk, put your things away and close the door. This is especially important if you work from home, so you can switch off and relax. Having work things hanging around into the evening means that the stress of the day will linger when you need to get some rest. Put your laptop away. Create a calm, clean space to return to tomorrow. You may want to signal the end of the working day with a ritual, such as lighting a candle or putting on a favourite tune.

CHAPTER THREE:

Stress-Free Evenings

Evenings are an essential time for rest and relaxation, connecting with friends and doing things that bring you joy. It's the time of day when you get to choose what you do, rather than just doing what you have to.

The tools and tips in this chapter are designed to help you wind down and prepare for a restful night's sleep. Lack of sleep can be a stressor in itself, so by helping yourself have a better night tonight, you are reducing your burden overall. Choose at least one tip from this chapter and do it this evening.

Your perfect evening

What does a perfect evening look like to you? There's no right or wrong answer to this, but it's worth thinking about so that you get the evening you want. Before you can create it, though, you need to be able to define it. What score out of ten, for relaxation, would you give your current typical evening? Are there any particular stressors in there, however small? If you could do whatever you wanted tonight, what would it be? Plan an evening that supports rather than drains you. Treat yourself to some precious and well-deserved relaxation time.

Rest is not a reward. It's a right. A requirement. Please stop waiting to rest until you have more time to do it.

KENDRA ADACHI

Gather the gold from today

As you move from daytime to evening, pause to take with you the good things about today. Ask yourself: What did I learn today? What can I take from today that's good?

You don't have to ignore the stressors of the day, but you can use them as a way to learn and move forwards in a more positive frame of mind. Ask yourself: What worked and what didn't work today? What filled me up and what emptied me out? What's the one thing I know for sure moving forwards?

Love yourself first and everything else falls into line. You really have to love yourself to get anything done in this world.

LUCILLE BALL

The 10-3-2-1 method for better sleep

Sleep experts recommend the 10-3-2-1 method as an easy way to get better-quality sleep.

- First, establish what time you intend to go to sleep. Then, working back from there:
- 10 hours before bed – no more caffeine.
- 3 hours before bed – no more big meals, so your body has a chance to rest and digest properly.
- 2 hours before bed – no more drinks, and also stop work and admin.
- 1 hour before bed – no screens. Put that phone away!

What you're doing with this approach is letting your body start to rest physically and mentally over an extended period of time. It takes less than a minute to consciously stop consuming drinks, food or digital content. Intentionally giving yourself a break from the work of digestion and mental stimulation means that when you do finally lie down and close your eyes, your body's already at least part of the way there. Easing your mind and body towards sleep in this way should result in a better-quality rest throughout the night.

Rest with repetitive movement

Repetitive, rhythmic movement shifts our minds into a calm, meditative state and can be particularly helpful for people dealing with chronic stress. Your evenings may be a more flexible time for hobbies and crafts, such as sewing, knitting, embroidery, colouring and jigsaws, which are all brilliant examples of coping mechanisms.

What type of repetitive physical movement would be fun for you? Maybe there's something you've already started and could pick back up? A small repetitive craft or hobby will give your mind a break from stress and make it better able to face tomorrow.

When we create peace and harmony and balance in our minds, we will find it in our lives.

LOUISE HAY

Five minutes of silence

It would be easy to fill your evening with entertainment, and you can still do that – but how about adding 5 minutes of silence for a change? Just quiet, just breathing. Netflix will still be there when you're done. Become more comfortable in your own thoughts. Get settled and still. After a busy day, your mind needs downtime. Give yourself the gift of a little pause of nothing.

No phone nights

Charging your phone outside of your bedroom is a small change that takes seconds to set up but will continue to benefit you as long as you do it. You'll be less likely to look at your phone last thing at night or first thing in the morning. Pinging notifications won't be able to interfere with your evening wind down. Checking messages, social media and emails late at night can impact sleep quality and leave us feeling more stressed and less rested. Make your bedroom your sanctuary from the stressors of the digital world.

Try gratitude journalling

Scientific studies have repeatedly found that people who regularly express gratitude experience lower levels of stress and improved well-being. In other words, if you pause to note the things that are good about your life, you will feel better for longer. And there's a particular benefit to making your gratitude practice an evening one. One study found that people who wrote down things they were grateful for at bedtime often slept better and woke up feeling more refreshed.

Why not make a short burst of gratitude journalling part of your night-time routine? Ask yourself: What am I thankful for that happened today? What am I grateful for right now in this moment?

If you're not into journalling, you could simply make a point of thinking about the things you're grateful for each evening. What three things do you want to say thank you for tonight?

TIMES OF STRESS ARE ALSO TIMES THAT ARE SIGNALS FOR GROWTH, AND IF WE USE ADVERSITY PROPERLY, WE CAN GROW THROUGH ADVERSITY.

ABRAHAM J. TWERSKI

Eat serotonin-boosting food

The food we eat has a big effect on how we feel, and some foods definitely help us be more positive, so try to include them in your evening meal. Certain foods can help increase serotonin levels (one of the brain's "feel-good" chemicals) because they contain tryptophan, an amino acid that converts into serotonin. Examples of foods that help with this are cheese, eggs, fish, milk, nuts, seeds (such as pumpkin seeds and sunflower seeds), tofu and turkey. What will you choose tonight?

Avoid blue light at night

Blue light is the part of the light spectrum that the human eye can see. When we get it from the sun, it helps us stay awake and can elevate our mood. However, too much blue light at night – from smartphones, computers and TV screens – can interfere with the production of melatonin, the hormone that helps us sleep. To avoid feeling stressed and tired, use dimmer lights in the evening and schedule your devices to automatically switch to night mode (or go offline entirely) so your brain gets the message that it's night-time.

Feelings come and go like
clouds in a windy sky.

THÍCH NHẤT HẠNH

Loving touch

Science has found that physical contact can really help with reducing stress hormones. Positive, gentle touch such as hugs, cuddles, a pat on the back or holding hands lowers the heart rate and blood pressure, which can be elevated if you've been stressed. Touch also triggers the release of oxytocin (known as the "love hormone"). Oxytocin helps reduce stress and promote feelings of calm and connection. And you don't have to wait for someone else to be around to enjoy the benefits of this type of contact – you can give it to yourself.

Tonight, make a point of taking care of your body as it has looked after you today. If you've been on your feet, maybe a foot massage or a hot bubble bath would be comforting. Try a facial or scalp massage, or deep-stretching any part of you that aches. Put on an overnight face mask to help rehydrate. Wear loose, comfortable clothes that feel good. Use the evening to reconnect with your body in a loving and positive way.

Sip a stress-free tea

Instead of caffeine, which will keep you awake, opt for a calming evening brew instead. Take your time and pause mindfully as your tea brews. Many brands offer special blends of sleep-friendly tea, or you could try:

- Camomile tea – known for its calming properties.
- Mint tea – to aid digestion after your evening meal.
- Valerian tea – valerian root has mild sedative qualities, so it's often used as a natural aid to relaxation.

The power of laughter

Nothing throws off the stress of the day like a really good belly laugh. It's the ultimate feel-good factor. Laughter has been found to decrease stress hormones and trigger endorphins to improve our mood. There are other physical health benefits as well – laughter boosts the immune system, helping our bodies fight off disease. Is there a TV show or podcast that's always guaranteed to tickle your funny bone? What's made you laugh recently? Will you make space for it tonight?

Laughter. An essential ingredient for survival.

PATTI SMITH

Prepare for morning

In the evening, get a jump-start on tomorrow by choosing your clothes and laying them out alongside anything else you might need. While you're at it, prepare for breakfast and lunch. This leaves you with fewer decisions to make in the morning, helps the start of the day flow more smoothly and allows you to be in less of a rush to get everything sorted. You're getting ahead of any potential stressors before they happen.

Relax your muscles

Progressive muscle relaxation (PMR) is a simple technique to take your body into a state of deep physical calm. As your body relaxes, so will your mind, as the parasympathetic nervous system is activated. If you're trying to get to sleep but you still feel tense from your day, PMR will help release those tensions and send you off into a blissful night's slumber.

It works by tightly clenching and then deeply relaxing each muscle group in the body in turn. Start at your toes and work your way up to your head (or vice versa if that feels better to you). Tense each muscle group in turn for around 5 seconds, then release for around 10 seconds. Don't rush. Take your time. Pay attention to how you feel as you relax, and the tension leaves your body. Enjoy slipping into a more tranquil state as, one by one, you tense, then let go of each set of muscles.

Let go, look forward

As part of letting go of the stresses of today, look towards tomorrow calmly. A new day is a blank page – a chance to start again. Spend a few minutes thinking or journalling about what's going on for you the following day. Create a clear picture in your mind of what you would be doing if you felt calmer tomorrow than you do today. What's the one thing you'd like to achieve tomorrow? This will help you feel more prepared and less likely to be dragged under by stress.

You must learn
to let go. Release the
stress. You were never
in control anyway.

STEVE MARABOLI

Make a plan

Get ahead of tomorrow's tasks by making a detailed list of what you need to do. What's on your agenda? Put some easy wins on there for things you'll be able to do and tick off quickly. This will give you a smoother jumping-off point from which to start the next day. Maybe add a little positive message to your future self who'll be reading this list in the morning. Your list will help you feel more in control of the demands of your day.

CHAPTER FOUR:

A Stress-Free Future

In this chapter, we're looking to stress-proof your future, to help you prevent stress when possible and deal with it more easily when it pops up.

You can utilize these tips for life to minimize the negative effects of stress in the long term. Some take a little longer to set up but will continue to benefit you on an ongoing basis. Choose one or two and commit to doing them this week. Claim your stress-free future by meeting it calmly, safe in the knowledge that you've got this.

Simplify your life

Physical and mental clutter go hand in hand, and both make life more stressful. Simplifying your life means your mind will have less to deal with, fewer choices to make and less stress as a result. Which part of your life could you simplify? Could you cut back on your commitments, clear the clutter from your bedroom or adopt a more streamlined wardrobe? Is there something you've been saying yes to, but now it's time to say no? Simplifying will mean fewer plates to spin, resulting in a less frazzled you.

Love lemonading

Scientists have found that taking a playful approach to life, aka "lemonading", helps boost resilience and will increase your ability to cope with stress. One study found that people who are more playful tend to be more optimistic and able to stay happy, in spite of life's challenges.

Fun, play, joy – they all deserve a daily place in your life. The more they fill your time, the more stress naturally gets squeezed to the side. And they're all there to be observed in the little moments: taking your favourite mug down off the shelf and remembering where you bought it; cuddling up with your pet; singing a silly song; climbing a tree; your wildest dance; a smile given or returned; good socks.

Be alert, alive, awake to the tiny moments of playful joy in your life today. Notice them, gather them, hold them close. And if life brings you lemons, try lemonading.

Adopting the right attitude can convert a negative stress into a positive one.

HANS SELYE

Wear stress-relief jewellery

Stress-relief jewellery is specifically designed to help the wearer feel more calm via sensory engagement – touch, sight, scent or all three. It's particularly useful if you want to keep your stress management private and portable. Nobody needs to know that your beautiful, beaded necklace is also helping you stay calm and focused, unless you want them to.

Practise radical acceptance

Radical acceptance means accepting your reality as it is, without judgement or attempting to change it. Even if life isn't going how you'd like it to right now, you can acknowledge it and make peace with it. At its heart, radical acceptance is about accepting yourself with compassion and love. Practising radical acceptance has been linked to a reduction in anxiety, depression and stress. By letting go of unrealistic expectations and learning to accept things as they are, you can cultivate a sense of inner peace and emotional resilience.

BE YOUR OWN
WORK IN PROGRESS...
YOU'RE A MASTERPIECE
IN THE MAKING.

DONNA ASHWORTH

Adopt a healthy routine

A structured (but flexible) routine based around self-care will help you deal with tough times when they come. By focusing on keeping yourself well, you'll become more resilient and less likely to burn out.

- Start the day calmly. The tips in chapter one will help you do this.
- Aim to eat nourishing foods as much as you can.
- Find a way to move that you enjoy and do it every day.
- Establish a night-time routine that leads towards sleep.

Don't try to reinvent your whole life at once. Think of your daily routine as the root that everything else grows from. Put self-care at the centre of your life, not as an optional add-on or extra. Stress will always come from somewhere, so get yourself in the best shape to deal with it.

Talk about how you feel

Stress is a normal part of everyone's life. There is not a person on the planet who ever existed who didn't have some sort of stress to deal with. Don't feel you have to keep yours to yourself – this is a part of human existence and it's good to share. If you're not comfortable talking about your stress to friends or family, consider speaking to a life coach, therapist or your doctor. You don't have to deal with this alone and the right people will be glad to help.

Create a calm soundtrack to your life

Whatever we decide to listen to has a direct effect on our mood, so make choices with calm in mind. Soft sounds can trigger a relaxation response and classical music is known to lower blood pressure. Is there a podcaster or audiobook narrator you like who has an incredibly soothing voice? Or is there calm chill-out music you particularly enjoy? You could even choose to listen to white noise or the sounds of nature. Create a soothing soundtrack that will put you in a more chilled frame of mind, and listen to it regularly.

Lean in to learning

When we learn something new, the brain releases dopamine (a "feel-good" hormone). Our minds focus on this new stimulation, naturally leading our thoughts away from any present stressors. Learning opens up our world, bringing in new stimuli and possibilities. It also brings a sense of accomplishment – that "yes, I can" feeling – giving a self-esteem boost.

You could learn something for fun, as a hobby, or because it will bring personal or work benefits. Feel more in control of your life by setting your own curriculum.

What would your future self be glad you started learning today?

Emotions are like passing storms, and you have to remind yourself that it won't rain forever.

AMY POEHLER

Monotask, not multitask

Multitasking can lead to overwhelm and burnout. It's far more restful for our brains to focus on one thing at a time, and not have to juggle lots of spinning plates at once. "Monotasking" is a form of mindfulness, helping us focus on the present moment only. Of course, in this busy, overstimulating world, that's easier said than done. Start small, and try to focus on doing one simple thing at a time, even if it's just making a cup of tea or taking a shower.

Minimize the number of tabs open when you're working on the computer. Turn off app notifications on your phone so they're not pinging, interrupting your focus. Aim to do one thing well, and to completion, rather than lots of half-baked things at once. Monotasking helps us be more present in our lives. The next thing you do, try to make sure it's that thing only.

The real character of men and women comes to the surface under stress.

LAURA INGALLS WILDER

Put nature where you'll see it

Nature is one of life's best de-stressors. Studies have found that even a picture of nature will be enough to unlock some of those de-stressing benefits. An easy way to integrate this tip into your life is to place images of or objects from nature wherever you often look. Set a picture of a beautiful outdoor scene as your phone's lock screen, or as the screen saver on your laptop. Place objects from nature on your desk or in your hallway. Access the power of nature even when life is keeping you indoors.

Stay connected with your circle

People enjoy being part of a community. Our network supports us and helps us see our own complicated lives in a wider context. While being alone and happy in your own company is a great skill to develop, we all benefit from having a mutually supportive community around us. Who do you spend most time with? Who is there in your life that makes you feel lifted when you spend time together? Who would you like to reconnect with that you haven't seen or talked to in a while? Contact at least one friend today and get a date in the diary to meet.

Let go of people who bring you down, and surround yourself with those who bring out the best in you.

TAYLOR SWIFT

Nurture your blue mind

Scientists have found that being in or around water helps us feel more relaxed, focused, happier and healthier. This is known as "Blue Mind" – the opposite of "Red Mind", which refers to feeling stressed and anxious.

Make spending time with water a priority – swim, walk by a lake, paddle in the ocean, visit a fountain. Pause, listen, be present and let the water help you feel restored.

Dear me...

Write a letter from your future, de-stressed self to you today. This is an act of creativity and imagination to keep you focused on the future you would like. It helps make the possibility of becoming that calm and peaceful person more real; that person who's no longer ground down by stress. What important story does your future, de-stressed self want to tell? What has your future self learned that you want to share? What helped you get to this version of yourself? What were the turning points? What did you leave behind? Explore this in a letter that's for your eyes only.

Make friends with your stress

A known situation is always much easier to deal with than something that's hovering in the background, threatening to happen. Facing up to your stress puts you in the driving seat. You're an active participant in your life, not just a victim. Stress is part of being human. And maybe even just that thought will help you feel more positive about the tough stuff you are facing. Remind yourself of the positive side of stress – it helps us get things done and rise to challenges. Change your thinking about stress and you will change your life.

YOU ARE YOUR BEST THING.

TONI MORRISON

Let go of what you can't control

Feeling in control (or not) is central to how we experience and deal with stress. We often experience stress because we feel that our lives are out of control. But ultimately, we are never totally in control of our lives anyway, so trying to be anything else is an impossible – and, yes, stressful – task. One big shift we can make that will transform our relationship with the stress in our lives, today, tomorrow, and always, is to let go of that which we can't control. This isn't about being passive or giving in to life's pressures. It's about accepting that there may be things going on that you can't change or predict the outcome of.

Instead, shift the focus to the parts of the picture you can control – your own feelings, reactions and behaviour. If there's a particular source of stress in your life, make two lists – write down the bits you can control and the bits you can't. Commit to letting go of the things you can't control and instead focus on the things you can. Trust yourself that you can and will navigate this stress.

Conclusion

The time you take to de-stress is never wasted. In fact, it's one of the most beneficial things you can do for yourself. Don't try to just power on through because you'll end up running on empty. Stress is a natural response to present danger. If you're stressed, you're not failing, you're just human. This is why our bodies and minds have evolved to deal with stress. You really have got this, in mind, body and soul.

You've already taken the first steps towards a more balanced life of less stress by picking up and reading this book. Now's the time to take it further. Which tips in this book spoke to you most clearly and would fit most easily into your life? That's the place to start. Take every opportunity you have to fill your life with calm – think of it as a deposit in the bank in case you need to draw on it in future. Learning to deal with stress effectively will reduce its negative impact and boost your everyday well being. Life doesn't have to be overwhelming. Claim calm as your birthright. Breathe. Move. Rise. Thrive.

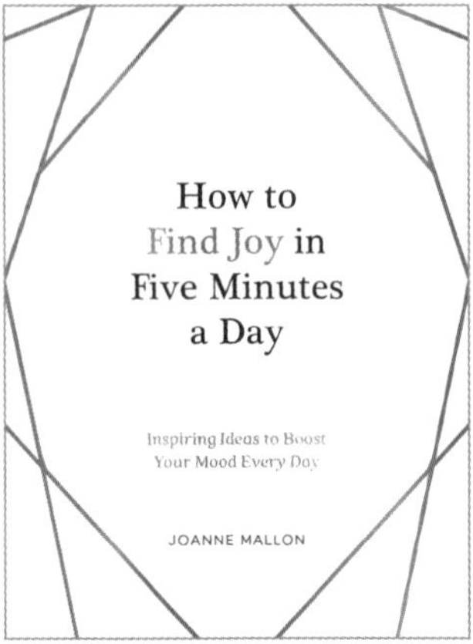

HOW TO FIND JOY IN FIVE MINUTES A DAY

Inspiring Ideas to Boost Your Mood Every Day

Joanne Mallon

Hardback

ISBN: 978-1-80007-156-8

This beautiful book includes tips and ideas to help you elevate your mood and liven up your routine. Perhaps you will try setting an intention, performing a small act of kindness, or eating outdoors in the fresh air. Even the smallest moment of positivity can transform your outlook, so whether you follow one tip or many, you are sure to lift your spirits and find a small oasis of happiness every day – all you need is five minutes.

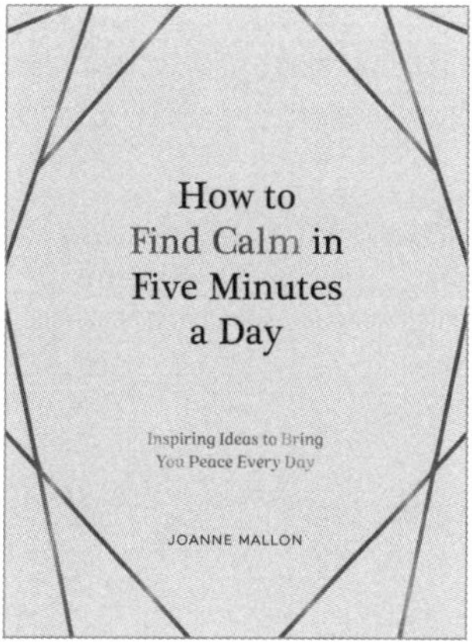

HOW TO FIND CALM IN FIVE MINUTES A DAY

Inspiring Ideas to Bring You Peace Every Day

Joanne Mallon

Hardback

ISBN: 978-1-83799-010-8

Pockets of calm are all around us, even on the busiest of days – and they're easy to find when you know where to look. All you need is five minutes. Guiding you through each stage of your day, these soothing rituals will help you recentre yourself and rise above everyday stresses.

Have you enjoyed this book?

If so, why not write a review on your favourite website?

If you're interested in finding out more about our books, find us on Facebook at Summersdale Publishers, on Twitter/X at @Summersdale and on Instagram, TikTok and Bluesky at @summersdalebooks and get in touch. We'd love to hear from you!

Thanks very much for buying this Summersdale book.

www.summersdale.com